Contents

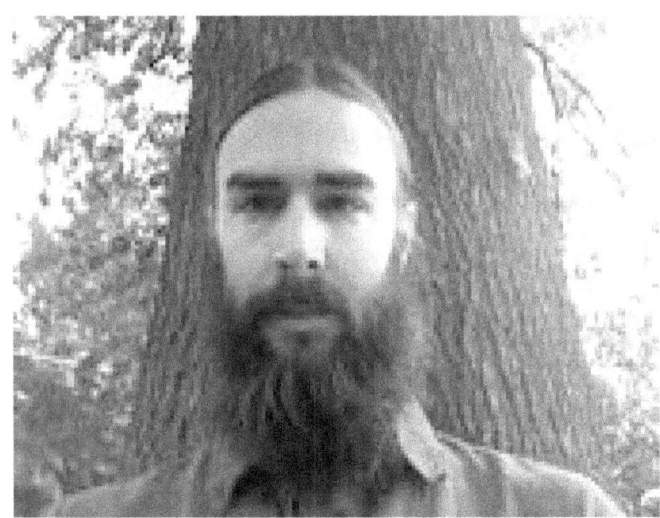

Andrew Bentley -Herbalist

This is Robert Rodgers from Parkinsons Recovery. I am currently in the clinic offices of Andrew Bentley who is a herbalist. It is a pleasure and delight to interview him today.

What is your background and how is it that you came to be an herbalist?

I grew up in a family and area where herbal medicine was used a lot and got started learning about it that way. Later I traveled around the world and studied with different traditional healers in different places and tried to learn how different cultures use the medicinal plants that grow in their areas.

I have been practicing since the mid 1990's and for the last 6 or 7 years I have also been doing some lecturing at the University of Kentucky medical school. I have also published various different papers on herbal medicine in scholarly journals and things of that nature. I have worked with lots and lots of patients.

Lexington is a relatively large city compared to other cities in Kentucky. Many people are not going to know a lot about what an herbalist does. How many herbalists are there in Lexington, Kentucky?

I am pretty much it as far as Lexington goes. I believe there is another herbalist practicing in Louisville and there are a few hundred of us throughout the country.

For somebody who has no clue, what does a herbalist do for people?

When someone comes into see me or when I am doing a phone consultation I get a lot of information from them and ask a lot of questions about both the specific issues they are having and their general background, their health, their lifestyle, their diet and so on.

What I try and do with all of that information is to figure out which structures and functions in their body are working adequately and which ones are not. Based on that I try and recommend herbs that will be helpful for that specific person in that specific situation to have those structures and functions work more appropriately.

If I were to talk with you today about some symptoms I am having, we would talk, you would ask me a lot of questions, then you might have some recommendations of herbs that I might take. Would I then take a prescription to a pharmacy that would be filled at the pharmacy or how exactly does that work?

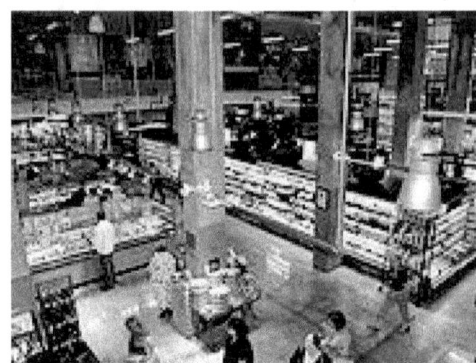

Like most herbalists I have a dispensary here in my clinic because not all of the herbs are readily available. If they were it would be possible to get them from a supplement store or health food store or someplace like that deals in herbal medicines. I try to keep everything I use on hand here so if I am using something unusual I can have it available for the person.

More specifically, you have seen many individuals with the symptoms of Parkinson's. Could you talk some about your observations in dealing with individuals who have the symptoms of Parkinsons?

Sure. My perspective involves less focus on a specific named disease entity and more focus on what is actually going on with the person's body. In people with these symptoms what we are usually seeing is a problem with the nervous system which can translate in to various different things coming up in other systems in the body because the nervous system is kind of the one in charge so to speak.

Problems result sometimes as a result of physical damage, sometimes as a result of drugs or other toxic substances. There are problems with the Substantia Nigra in the brain and problems with the production and

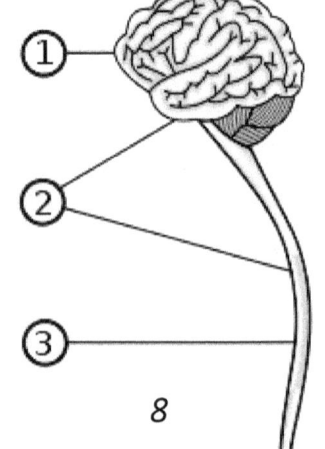

uptake of <u>dopamine</u> in the nervous system, particularly in the <u>central nervous system</u>.

My focus in terms of working with these individuals is to try and support the functioning of the nervous system and particularly the functions by which the <u>dopamine</u> channels work in the <u>central nervous system</u>.

People are always on the lookout for particular ways to do that or particular herbs that can support those types of systems.

What <u>herbs</u> in your past experience are helpful for people who have central nervous system challenges?

There are certainly a lot of them and exactly which ones are appropriate include a lot of things that are going on with the person, including what sort of events might have precipitated the start of the symptoms.

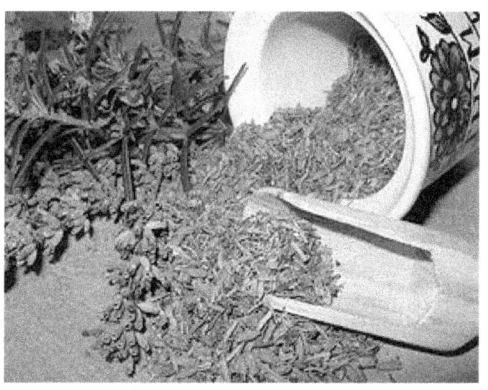

For example, sometimes you will see Parkinsonian type situations that are a result of trauma. Other times it is maybe hereditary or we do not know where it came from. Maybe it is something that has come about as a slow process rather than something suddenly.

In all cases there is more or less something amounting to physical damage in the nervous system.

There are certain things that are fundamentally helpful with getting the nervous system to repair itself. One of the things I use in that capacity is an herb called Bacopa. Bacopa comes to us from the traditional medicine of India. As such it has a very long documented history of use for helping the nervous system repair itself.

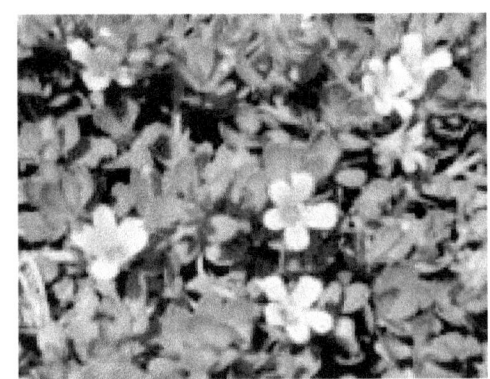

Most of the herbs I use are a liquid extract and it is one that I use in that way. That can sometimes help. There are a few other herbs that help along those same lines that help with actually physically repairing the tissue in the nervous system. There are others ones that help to change the chemistry of the nervous system.

A good example of that is Barley Malt Extract. It is a particular extract prepared from barley malt that contains a substance called Hordenine which has a very strong effect on the dopamine pathways in the brain.

There are some other things that may help on a more symptomatic level or help more with the peripheral nervous system. For example Oat Straw extract helps to calm the tremors that most people have.

Valerian can also be helpful in that capacity sometimes.

There are several different categories of herbs that help with different functions and different structures in the body and in the nervous system. In each of those categories there are many different herbs that might be helpful depending on the particular individual.

Robert: As I understand it then, it really depends on what the symptoms are that are presenting that would inform which herbs you would recommend the person begin taking.

If a person came in and had a dominate tremor, that would inform a certain set of herbs or maybe just one dominate herb versus if someone came in with a dominate symptom of pain and rigidity, that would inform a different recommendation of herbs. Do I understand this correctly?

Yes that is right. It depends on the presenting systems and to a certain extent which category of herbs we are choosing. Which herbs we are choosing depends a lot on the body type of the particular person and that person's constitution and make up.

If someone has a lot of tremors then something that is an anti-spasmodic might help more than if someone is experiencing a lot of pain and rigidity, in which case we might use an entirely separate type of things. Some things are helpful more or less across the board.

_For example, the _Barley Malt extract_ is one that actually helps with the levels of dopamine in the brain which is almost always amiss in Parkinson's disease because of the nature of the condition. That is_ *something that is usually helpful. It still depends on the person and what other therapies the person might be taking.*

For example, if someone were taking dopamine or Levodopa, I probably would not use that herb. It might increase the amount of those or decrease the clearance of those substances because then you start seeing things which are not really the goal. It depends on a lot of things but definitely the presenting symptoms are a very big factor in choosing which herbs to choose.

Robert: The bottom line is that people who decided to listen to this interview hoping that you were going to give them a particular list of herbs that they could take to feel better are not going to get that list. It is really idiosyncratic to the individual. It depends on exactly what is going on with the individual. I do have many people who ask very specific questions because the symptoms for Parkinsons are so varied.

Many people ask me a question about excessive salivation. They have a lot of worries and troubles with that. Is there anything off the top of your head that you would suggest as a possibility in the herbal area for that?

There are some things that might help with that. For example, oak bark extract taken in very small amounts can sometimes help with excessive salivation. Also sometimes if you have better muscle control in the muscles of the neck and throat and the face, that can sometimes help for the excessive salivation not to be a problem.

As far as the herbs go, although there is no one size fits all list, I would definitely be glad to talk about specific herbs more and say which ones I would use and under what circumstances they are helpful.

You mentioned people with tremors. I had mentioned oat straw as one thing that is sometimes helpful for that. A nice thing about oat straw is that it usually does not cause drowsiness. A lot of things that are anti-spasmodic also cause sedation. Sometimes people aren't looking for that. That is a helpful thing about that particular herb because it doesn't have so much of that effect.

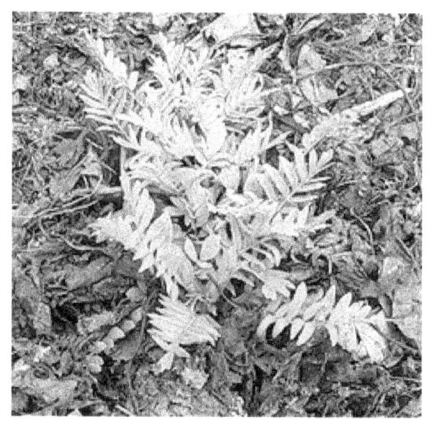

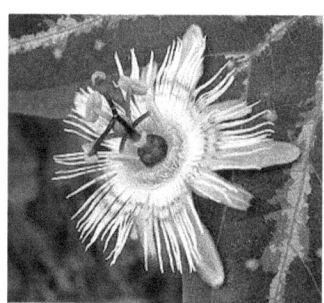

Valerian is a much stronger herb for helping to suppress tremors but it does carry some risk of sedation, of feeling more drowsy and so forth especially when people first start taking it. Sometimes that lessons as time goes on. It is a very strong substance when it comes to helping control involuntary muscle movement tremors and involuntary movement of otherwise involuntary muscles. It is a good one for that.

Passion flower is also one that is helpful for some particular individuals. These are all things that would go into that category of working on tremors.

As far as rigidity goes, one of my favorite things for that is an herb called Artemisia or sometimes it is called wormwood. That is a herb that helps the mechanism by which the nerve impulses are transmitted in the body. It is very good for rigidity of all sorts including what sometimes accompanies Parkinson's. So that is something I use both as an extract.

There is also a procedure that is done with it called Moxibustion. We have these rolled up sticks of crushed Artemisia leaf which are lit and held near basically acupuncture points. They affect the flow of energy in the body. That can sometimes help with some of these same types of things – with tremors as well as rigidity actually.

see

is

What people cannot see is that you are actually holding a device for me so I was able to see what it looks like. When you are saying you put that on various acupuncture points in the body, this something you do for people when they come to see you or is this something you teach people how to for themselves?

For the most part I do use it as an office procedure. Most acupuncturists also use Moxibustion (which is the name of the procedure). People do it different ways.

Sometimes I do teach people where specific points are, but which ones are helpful is different depending on what part of someone's body they are having trouble with.

There are certain meridians, certain lines on the body, on the face, on the arms, on the trunk of the body, on the legs that are relevant points within those meridians.

In the way I use Moxibustion it is not actually applied to the skin. It is just held near the skin so that it warms it without actually burning the skin. Some people do actually practice a style of Moxibustion where they blister the skin. I do not do that. For one thing it hurts and people don't like it. For another, there are also risks of infection and slow healing and so forth.

This device looks a bit like a very large and long cigarette with a gold cap on one end. You light it on the other end. It does look like it would hurt if you applied it directly to the skin.

Some people write me questions about depression who have the symptoms of Parkinson's. What would be recommendations for a person who presents that as a primary symptom?

I think the two are really closely related. The chemistry of depression and the chemistry of   Parkinson's are very similar.

One involves *serotonin*.

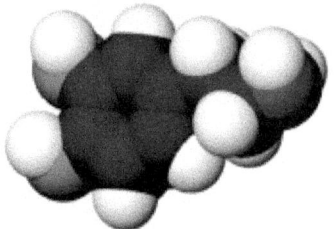

The other involves *dopamine*.

Other than that they are virtually identical.

One herb I use a lot of is *Saint John's Wart* which is also known as *Hypericum* That is something you can get at almost any health food store. It works kind of slowly, but it does have a tendency to work pretty well a lot of the time.

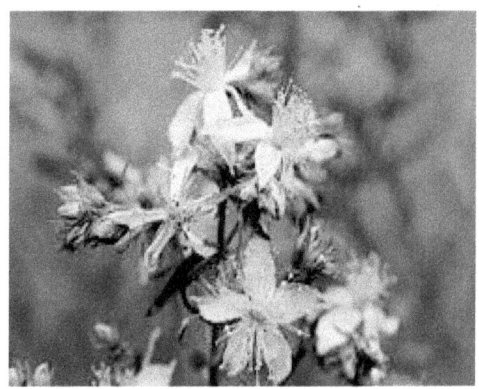

Basically it does a number of things. One of the things that has been most researched is that it helps to increase the amount of *serotonin* in the brain which is good.

It also helps to clear toxins from the body, all sorts of different toxins and substances.

For some people with Parkinson's that is very relevant. For some people that herb will actually make a pretty big difference in how they are feeling from day to day; in other people, not so

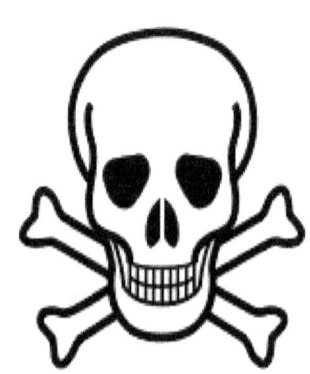

much. It is a good first line herb for supporting the nervous system for someone who is depressed.

There is also the <u>Artemisia</u> which I previously mentioned is pretty strongly anti-depressant as well when taken internally. That is another one I might use in that situation. Depression takes a lot of different forms in a lot of different people as well. Those are some of the most common things that I use most frequently.

After a person sees you and you provide them with the herbs that occur to you would be helpful, you give specific recommendations on how much of that herb to take. So, you prescribe one teaspoon, one drop or one whatever. Is that correct?

Yes, that is right. The amounts I use tend to be quite a bit larger than the amounts that are usually recommended if you go and buy a bottle of the stuff from a health food store.

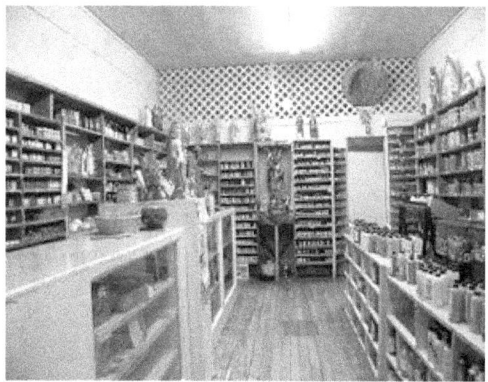

Then again it is under professional supervision so there is a little more control and more ability to look out for things that might not be desired outcomes.

I give people recommendations on how much to take and when to take it. Then, I usually follow up with the person in about a week or so and see what has changed – if anything has changed that quickly.

At that point a lot of what I am trying to see is whether they are tolerating the treatment. A couple weeks down the road we can get a clearer picture of whether the treatment is working well. With certain herbs like the Barley Malt – I have definitely had times when people came to see me in a wheel chair and were able to walk out because it makes a big difference pretty quickly in how their nervous system is functioning. It can be the difference between having a good day and having a bad day or having a lot of good days and a lot of bad days.

In the process of working with clients it is in part a question of experimentation. You start with a particular set of prescriptions with one or several herbs. The person takes it and then comes back with reports on how they are doing. There is then follow up with perhaps some adjustments of those as a function of how their symptoms have shifted. Is that right?

Yes. That is basically right. I wish I was smart enough to always get it right the first time but I am not and I do not think anyone else is either. There is definitely some room for trying it out and seeing what works with a particular person. Maybe the dose is not strong enough or maybe it is producing some other outcome that we do not want.

For example, I mentioned that drowsiness can be produced by some of the same things that produce tremors. We look out for those kinds of things. Sometimes you have to adjust the dosages. Sometimes you have to adjust what the person is taking. It is work.

It is a process that sometimes takes some time. It is possible to get everything right in the beginning but it often takes a bit of working with it. Usually from the beginning of treatment people can tell that something is going on even if it is not exactly the outcome they were looking for.

Parkinsons Recovery is all about hope, giving people hope that it is possible to get some relief from their symptoms. You have given a few hints that one of the reasons I am here in Lexington talking with you today in your clinic is that the work you have done with people who have Parkinsons is providing relief from their symptoms.

Could you talk about your experience with people who have the symptoms of Parkinsons and how these herbs have helped them?

Usually what I see is some fairly immediate reduction of symptoms. Sometimes people are able to get where they are more or less symptom free or have a very livable amount of symptoms. Sometimes people don't have any appreciable symptoms at all and are maybe even able to stop taking the herbs.

There is the actual potential for healing, for the body to actually get itself back into the state it is supposed to be in rather than just relying on supplementation and on other things to keep it going. That can be different from one person to the next certainly. Strangely enough, it is not always related to how bad their symptoms are in the first place.

I mentioned in talking about the Barley Malt, the Hordenine that I have seen people go from not being able to walk because they are having very severe tremors and rigidity to being able to walk in a fairly short amount of time. That represents a very immense change in quality of life.

What I am mostly going for is change in quality of life. I am not at all concerned with figures and numbers and test results. I am really concerned with the subjective reports of

> *"How are you feeling?"*

> *"Is it better than before we started this?"*

That tends to be what I work towards.

It sounds like for the people with Parkinson's that you have seen the results are indeed encouraging. People are seeing relief from their symptoms. You offer hope that there are people who have become virtually symptom free – maybe not totally – but virtually symptom free. Do I understand that correctly? Is that what you said?

Yes, that is what I said. Certainly that is an atypical result. I am not going to promise that happens for everybody by any means. I think a lot of it depends on how determined people are and how hard they work for it and what steps they are willing to take.

Certainly most people I have seen that have had the most success have used a variety of different treatments, not just what I am doing, but also maybe conventional treatment, what I am doing and acupuncture. There are various other things people do. I think there is definitely room for all of them to work together in a single person's body. Yes. Sometimes I have seen results that are really, really good. Of course, that is what everybody wants to see.

You are a very modest man and basically what you are reporting is that many people who are seeing significant improvement in symptoms are seeing other people and doing other things. You are not able to attribute the actual work of the herbs exclusively as the primary cause of their getting better. The fact is that clearly the herbs are playing a role as well. That is incredibly hopeful, especially in a situation where many people who get the symptoms of Parkinson's believe that they are always going to get worse. What you are saying is no, no, that is not true in your experience.

Do people get worse that you have seen as patients?

I have seen people get worse. So far, I do not think I have had anybody I have worked with where we were not able to turn that around. It is the normal course of the condition to get worse in a lot of cases. Sometimes that is still happening.

My goal is always to halt and reverse that downward progress. I believe that the herbs facilitate or make room for the process of healing that is built into the body.

Years ago people used to say that damage to the central nervous system is permanent. Period. There is no way that this tissue can ever regenerate. If it is damaged - if it is in a bad state - there is no way it is ever going to get better.

That is antiquated information at this point. We now know that is not always the case. We have always had stories of people where that did not happen to be the case.

It is now pretty well accepted in the world of physiology that central nervous tissue can regenerate itself even in an adult, but that it often doesn't. My goal in terms of that is to:

1. *Facilitate the healing process that is really an innate part of what the body is supposed to do.*

2. *Give the body the tools, the nourishment and the substances that it needs to do that process of healing.*

Robert: So, what you are saying is that the body knows how to heal itself. The herbs are facilitating that innate wisdom. Is that right?

Yes. That is my experience and my interpretation of what is going on.

I am sitting here with Andrew and behind him are three rows of many, many bottles of herbs and various concoctions. It is very clear that these bottles were not purchased at the supermarket down the street. Could you say something about where all these exotic looking herbs come from?

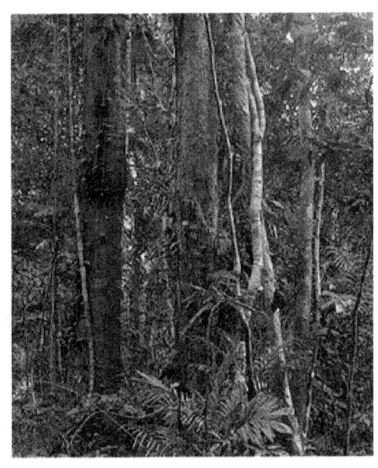

Most of them are wild. For the most part I use things that grow in the wild because they have to be strong. They have to contain the substances in strong amounts to be able to survive. Most of what I have I gather from the wild. A small percentage of it is stuff that I have grown for me by organic farmers. That would

apply to things that won't grow in the environment that I live in.

I have some things – for example, the <u>*Frankincense*</u> *- is grown in the* <u>*Arabian Peninsula*</u> *on an organic farm. I buy it from the people who grow it rather than trying to grow* <u>*Frankincense*</u> *in Kentucky which won't work. For the most part they are wild. The ones that are not wild are organically grown.*

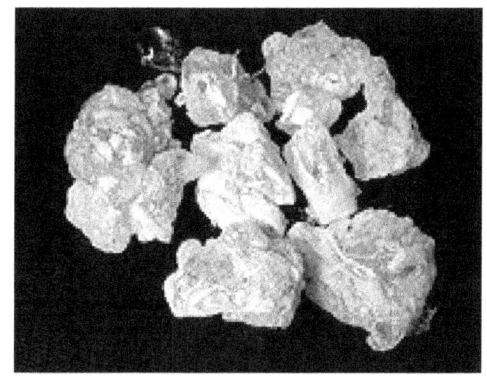

I just want to make sure that there is not even the faintest trace of contamination. I like to make sure I know where every bit of medicine I give to my patients has been from the time it was a seed growing until the time it is a finished product that I am handing to them.

Robert: What an amazing answer.

As I understand it, when you say they grow in the wild you actually go to places, identify the plants and harvest the plants yourself. Do I understand that correctly?

Yes. Most of them I harvest myself. I do have other people that do some harvesting for me, people I know that I can trust. Once I get the plant I am able to look at it both microscopically and visually and make sure it is exactly what I want it to be and that it is a good specimen of what I want it to be and it is not something that has sat on the shelf for years or something like that.

We have many people who are listening to and reading this interview who live far distant from Kentucky, many people from

many other countries. How would they be able to get assistance from you? Can they get a phone consultation from you and get some help in that way?

I can do phone consultations. It is always better if I have the person in front of me because I can actually look at them and so forth. When I actually examine somebody I can get some more information.

If people can make the trip I think that is better. Obviously that is not an option for everybody. I think it is good to do phone consultations also. I am available for that.

I can ship these herbs pretty much anywhere in the world. I have patients all over the place that I do that with sometimes. That is definitely a possibility.

I may be able to refer someone to a local herbalist. There are certainly all qualities of herbalists out there in the world, but there are some very good ones in a lot of places that people could get similar advantages from working with.

What is the phone number that people can reach you at?

My phone number is 859-420-5648. I can also work with people by e-mail. My e-mail address is Bentley@consultant.com

Is there a website?

I have a Myspace page where I put all my writings about herbal medicine. That is at www.myspace.com/kyherbalist

You mentioned you would be happy to connect people up with a herbalist in their area. Is there some listing of herbalists or some association that would have lists of individuals that would have your similar training?

Unfortunately no. There is not at this point. Hopefully that situation will be remedied in the future.

One specific herb that I do not think you have mentioned (and what many people are interested in) is called Mucuna Many people have been acquiring that from India as a dopamine supplement. Do you have any experience with that particular herb?

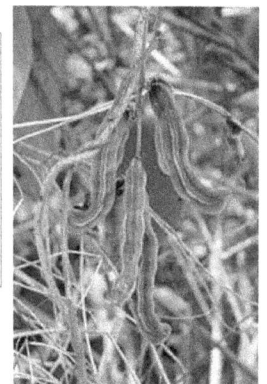

A little bit. I have worked with some people that have been using it. I personally really do not have a source for it at present so I haven't been using it.

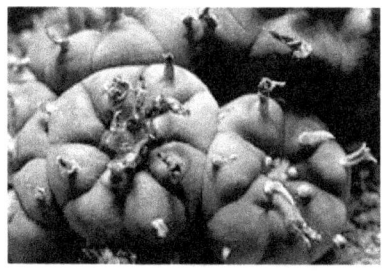

I think that in terms of how it works it is fairly similar in terms of outcome at least to the Hordenine or to the Peyote Cactus which is sometimes used.

I use the Barley Malt for something similar as far as raising the amount of dopamine in the central nervous system. It is something that is very easy to produce. It doesn't rely on anything exotic.

It is basically just barley, but the barley is spouted and prepared in a certain way. The Mucuna or the Levodopa have similar outcomes in terms of what they do to the chemistry of the central nervous system.

> **You have mentioned the Barley Malt several times. Is that something that people might be able to purchase at a health food store?**

Not that I am aware of actually. It is a traditional remedy that goes back to ancient Greece, probably older than that. At least Grecians were the first people that wrote about their experiences with Barley Malt.

I am not aware of it being sold as a supplement. I think one reason for that is that if you took too much, it would cause hallucinations, disorientation and things like that. It is pretty self limiting. You would not want it to happen while you were driving or operating heavy machinery or anything like that. It is not physiologically dangerous.

I don't think very many manufacturers would be willing to just put that on the shelves of health food stores because of the potential for liability if someone decides they are going to take the whole bottle of it and has a bad experience.

> **Everything we have talked about are herbals. They do not require (certainly in Kentucky) in most states or countries a prescription from a medical doctor. Is that correct?**

That is right. In the United States herbal medicines are regulated as dietary supplements which means they are not considered food or drugs. They are sort of an in between category.

There are manufacturing practices in place now. There is not quite the same pre market testing required that there is of drugs. There is that issue.

Sometimes quality control can be an issue which is why I have my own dispensary here. That is something that has improved by leaps and bounds over recent years. Then again, some of the things I have mentioned, particularly the Barley Malt, are not readily available as a supplement as far as I am aware of.

Some of these herbs do have side effects. It is important then for a person who wants to pursue this for themselves to consult with somebody such as yourself who is an expert on what the herb can do for them and also on possible side effects.

That is right and this is especially true if someone is already taking prescription drugs that it might interact with. There are cases where an herb and a drug with similar activities will counter act each other and basically amount to nothing. There are also instances where the two of them might do more than what is desired in any given direction taken together.

There are certainly things that can happen, things to look out for with particular herbs that might mean you are getting too much. Everyone's level of dosage that their body will respond to and tolerate is a little bit different with herbs as with any other substance.

This has been a fascinating discussion. I want you to know Andrew I feel like I have searched all over the country for you and finally found you. It is obvious that your skills, your abilities, your talents and your revelations with regard to what really helps people with the symptoms of Parkinson's are remarkable.

I want to thank you for providing your expertise, your knowledge, your insights and your advice to people with regard to herbals that might be used to help with the symptoms of Parkinson's. We have a Teleseminar series where people can ask guests questions that they have about various subjects. Could I twist your arm and encourage you to do a Teleseminar with me for people with Parkinson's at some point in the near future?

I would be glad to have the opportunity to do that.

Thank you so much. And I want to say thank you so much for doing this interview. This has been absolutely, totally amazing.

Index